THE PRONUNCIATION PART

Flavian Mark Lupinetti

Winner of The Poetry Box® Chapbook Prize 2024

Editing & Book Design by Shawn Aveningo Sanders
Cover Design & Artwork by Robert Sanders
    (RobertSandersCreative.com)

The Pronunciation Part
Winner, The Poetry Box® Chapbook Prize 2024
(Selected by Donna Hilbert)

ISBN: 978-1-956285-79-6
Published in the United States of America
Wholesale Distribution by Ingram Group

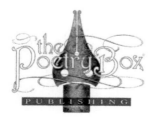

Published by The Poetry Box®, February 2025
Portland, Oregon, United States
website: ThePoetryBox.com

Every surgeon carries within him a little cemetery,
where from time to time he goes to pray,
a cemetery of bitterness and regret, in which
he seeks the meaning for certain of his failures.

—Rene Leriche

CONTENTS

Doctor Ruiz didn't quit his job today

but he must have thought about it
when we came in for our morning shift,
and Jim, who pulled nights this week,
signed out the ICU patients—
eight on ventilators, ten stable off them,
six who could go either way.
Oh, and Mrs. Bowen,
the one you intubated yesterday?
She boxed last night.

I bet he thought about it again
when the coding clerk
asked him to revise
his progress notes on Mrs. Bowen,
whom he'd taken care of for a month.
Can you add more diagnoses?
the clerk asked.   *For accuracy.*
Doctor Ruiz translated:
For jacking up the reimbursement.

Maybe he thought about it again
when he intubated Room 23.
I asked, *Is that the guy?*
and we both knew who I meant—
the guy who didn't practice distancing,
the guy who said only pussies wear masks,
the guy who learned that Doctor Ruiz
was a Dr from the DR and from then on
referred to Doctor Ruiz as Sammy Sosa.

I know he thought about it
when he told me over lunch,

[. . .]

This place treats us like the fucking janitors.
I showed him the Espada poem,
the one about the janitor who quit his job.
He said, *Write a poem about me.*
Call it Doctor Ruiz finally quits.

Yet I can tell all thoughts
of quitting are forgotten
by the time our twelve hours end
and we drag ass out to the garage.
Last year nights like this
we went home and texted each other
while watching Cubs highlights.

But this is the spring of 2020.
There may be no baseball this season,
only the virus is catching,
and the only ones I know for sure
will step up to the plate tomorrow
are me and Doctor Ruiz.

I Accompany My Old High School Teammate, Gino, to His First Round of Chemo

How calmly you awaited the test results that would determine
whether you got treated or whether this was a wasted trip.
How nonchalant when informed of the abundance of your white
  blood cells.
And your red ones. And your platelets, praise their presence,
they showed up for the party, too.

I warned you not to ask for tuna on whole wheat from Dorothy,
who pushes the cart around this grand ballroom,
and when you did anyway, you could have skipped the editorial
  comment.
She did not operate the machine that creates the feeble gray
  exudate
that smells like it came from Jiffy Lube,
nor did she inject it between the starchy beige planks, so you
need not have asked whether she knows this stuff can kill you.
Jesus, she's a volunteer.
After you get finished, we'll go to Whole Foods
for your gourmet pâté and your designer bread.

See the people sitting in the comfortable recliners like you?
Many have the same every-three-week schedule you do.
That means you'll see a lot of the same faces.
Then one week, you'll notice an absence.

Not wearing your usual muscle shirt, proud as you are
of having kept up, unlike me, the weight routine
Coach Kovalick imposed upon us half a century ago?
The port dangling below your clavicle embarrasses you.
Still, next time don't wear that turtleneck.
Make it easier on the nurses.

[. . .]

The pharmaceuticals take time to achieve
their pyrrhic victory, laying waste to the misbehaving cells
while inflicting collateral damage on your
follicles, fingertips, cuticles, nerve endings.
Many people take advantage of the discomfort, however mild,
and the anxiety, however severe, to ask the nurse for good drugs.
Don't play the tough guy. You've earned the narcs and benzos,
fair recompense for the goddamn tuna.

It took an hour and a half to complete the infusion.
It will take an hour and a half every time.
Do not expect that with practice you can speed up the process.

You were gracious in thanking the nurse who unplugged you
and the clerk who gave you a return appointment
and the chaplain who offered to pray for you.
Despite yourself you found him charming for his sincerity
and good intentions, and I believe you charmed him when you said,
"Don't squander your intercessionary efforts on my atheist ass.
Save your ammunition for world peace, or someone's SAT scores,
or at least a football game."

Rejection Speech

that you can't trust a teenager
is a lesson I learned the hard way
because I trusted Tommy who was
thirteen when I met him but with
the physique of a four-year-old
thanks to a heart the size of a
half deflated beachball and just as robust
when it came to pumping blood and
although some of my colleagues said
he was too sick for me to do anything
I transplanted his heart and
by the following spring he played
Little League—not well; it turns out
that hitting a curve ball can't
be transplanted—and over the
following years he took his antirejection
drugs and made his appointments
and developed a side hustle talking
to civic groups to raise money
for the hospital until five years later
when he decided taking meds
sucked so he quit taking them
(rejection, obituary) and if Tommy
was the only teenager who did this
that would be tragic enough but Charlene
age fourteen did the same thing because
the drugs grew hair on her forehead
and her back—talking Lon Chaney
wolfman pelt here—and Derek at sixteen
moved out of his mom's house
to live in the trunk of a friend's car
before giving up and that shit happens

[. . .]

over and over and over so don't say a
fucking word to me when I transplant
kids who are mentally challenged
because one thing I can count on is
they're supervised so closely they never
miss a dose and the other thing I can
count on is I never have to ask myself
should I have put that heart into somebody else

Velocity Squared

After the gun smoke clears
the EMTs bring the victims to my ER,
and I ask them why they bothered,
and they say you need to pronounce them,
so I perform the only function I am capable of
under these circumstances—the pronunciation part—
Dead . . . Dead . . . Dead . . . Dead . . .
because an AR-15 transforms human bodies
into gobbets of protoplasm resembling
pathology specimens more than people,
consistent with the law of physics that decrees
force equals one half mass times velocity squared.

After the gun smoke clears,
I reflect on the ingenuity of Eugene Stoner,
who cleverly designed his AR-15 to fire
rounds of a petite .223 caliber but to propel
them at 3200 feet per second, because
how else do you penetrate steel plate at 500 yards
or disarticulate a leg from the pelvis
with a flesh wound below the knee
unless you rely on velocity squared?

After the gun smoke clears,
I stare in amazement at these headless corpses
and exploded chests, each resulting
from a single shot, yet mathematically
the calculations are correct:
to create an exit wound the
size of a cantaloupe with a bullet
smaller around than your Bic pen,
you gotta have that velocity squared.

Any Port in a Storm

My mental dictionary
has reordered its definitions
of the word *port*,
demoting to second
the entry describing
the post-prandial sip,
the rich and now forbidden fruit,
to third a town with a harbor,
to fourth a nautical direction—
right or left, I can never
keep them straight—
allowing definition number five
to carry port the verb.
Starting today, port
in the prime position denotes
this novel addition to my anatomy,
what the nurse impales with the needle
to send the poison pouring
through my veins.

I dreamed last night
of my port migrating
from under my clavicle
to the back of my neck,
metamorphosizing
from a fluid linkage
to a USB interface,
enabling the nurse
to scour my hard drive
of corrupt files,
download the fix,
and remove all the malware.

Samuel L. Jackson Pulls a Shift in the ICU at the Height of the Pandemic

motherfucker in Room Eleven
turning blue around the gills
intubate the motherfucker
ten more hours in my shift

turning blue around the edges
week old donuts in doctors' lounge
nine more hours in my shift
can Dunkin make a ventilator?

doctors' donuts down disposal
my home-made mask is one week old
can anyone make a ventilator?
I wonder if I can get the test

my home-made mask is one week old
starting to grow a greenish coating
I wonder if I fail the test
I wonder if I can smash my pager

Room Eleven's started coding
left a list of next of kin
gave them the number of my pager
Jesus Christ I hope they lost it

don't have time to call the kin
motherfucker in Room Eighteen
Jesus Christ he's gonna lose it
intubate the motherfucker

Surgery Interns Know the Rules

never let anyone see
how scared you are

if anybody asks you if you've
done one of these before
you say yes I've done one
because no one wants
to take responsibility
for helping you do your first
but if you say you've done several
you might not get the help you need

never say oops
always say there

nobody grades you anymore
on a scale from A to F
henceforth those who judge your
performance do so on a spectrum
with Bugs Bunny at one end
and Elmer Fudd at the other

there's one bad thing about
in house call every other night—
you miss half the good stuff

some of your mentors operate
at the speed of light
others at the speed of dark
you can do nothing about this

if you need help managing a sick patient
calling someone more experienced—
a senior resident, an attending—
will always be regarded
as a sign of weakness

the only clue the patient has
about the quality of the surgery
is how well you closed the skin

Operating Theater

When I give the order to start   the pump, and the maimed
heart muscle collapses like the rotten   rubber of a busted out two-ply tire,

I face the possibility that my meager vein grafts won't get this patient
out of the room alive. He could die on the table, right in front of me.

Or he might succumb later tonight, following a brief struggle. Or
linger a few days more, until my siege of drugs and machines

and consultant opinions prove futile. The answers must
await the climax of the operation and the denouement.

When I think about this stage, these special effects,
and the remote possibility of a happy ending,

I wonder why it took me so long to grasp the
meaning of the words *Operating Theater*.

In this drama I play two roles,
protagonist and spectator,

actor who does not
know the ending,

audience member
who cannot find
the exit.

The Anatomy Lesson of Doctor Nicolaes Tulp

On an unseasonably warm day in January of 1632
Aris Kindt made his dramatic debut before
a capacity crowd at the Waaggebouw in Amsterdam.
Hanged only a few hours earlier for petty thievery,
Kindt was an obvious choice for the lead
given his youth and absence of obvious pathology.
Nobody else auditioned.

Directed by Doctor Nicolaes Tulp, doyen of Anatomy,
whose cadaveric dissections had become an annual
spectacle, Kindt offered a unique interpretation of the role.
Instead of the traditional abdominal opening
for extraction of the gastrointestinal system,
Kindt's dismemberment began with the limbs.

Tulp's production proved a great success with
both the Guild of Surgeons, members of which
crowded closely to observe the anatomic minutiae,
and with the paying customers, members of the
aristocracy and the mercantile elite, proud of
their city's claim to world leadership in
advancing from the Dark Ages into a new
era of Light.

So pleased was Tulp by the performance
and by the attentive sketches Rembrandt
made during the show that he never noticed
the old master's mistake in the final painting,
incorrectly portraying the dissected left hand
as possessing the anatomy of the right.

Or did Rembrandt truly nod?

[. . .]

Art historians speculate that
this discrepancy may have been intentional,
Rembrandt's silent protest to show his abhorrence
at the annihilation of Aris Kindt.

The banquet that followed was said
to be most felicitous as well.
History does not record
who carved the roast.

Black Box Trilogy

By law, prescription medications come with package inserts that list possible side effects. The scariest and most dangerous side effects appear surrounded by a black box. These erasure poems are distilled from package inserts that include Black Box Warnings.

Your doctor has never read a Black Box Warning.

1. A Basketball Parent's Meditation

High potential?
Attention should be paid.
Volunteers are active.
A minor can be normal.

The presence must be
accounted for:
—poor follow through
—poor effort

Hostility?
There is no hostility.
Children who rebound
will be monitored.

Difficulties with agents?
Agents are inhibited by
slow poisoning.
I should know.
Elimination in 14 hours
can result.

Tell your child you are suspicious.
Tell your child you are not real.
Tell your child you are very anxious.
Tell your child, "You need to be adjusted."

What is most important?
Heart.
Height.
Vision.
Ability to drive.

Source: Package insert for Adderal (dextroamphetamine, legal speed)

~

Adderall® tablets contain d-amphetamine and l-amphetamine salts in the ratio of 3:1. Following administration of a single dose 10 or 30 mg of Adderall® to healthy **volunteers** under fasted conditions, peak plasma concentrations occurred approximately 3 hours post-dose for both d-amphetamine and l-

~

hydroxyamphetamine, or on the side chain α or β carbons to form alpha-hydroxy-amphetamine or norephedrine, respectively. Norephedrine and 4-hydroxy-amphetamine **are** both **active** and each is subsequently oxidized to form 4-hydroxy-norephedrine. Alpha-hydroxy-amphetamine undergoes

~

CYP2D6 is genetically polymorphic, population variations in amphetamine metabolism are **a** possibility.

Amphetamine is known to inhibit monoamine oxidase, whereas the ability of amphetamine and its metabolites to inhibit various P450 isozymes and other enzymes has not been adequately elucidated. In vitro experiments with human microsomes indicate minor inhibition of CYP2D6 by amphetamine and **minor** inhibition of CYP1A2, 2D6, and 3A4 by one or more metabolites. However, due to the probability of auto-inhibition and the lack of information on the concentration of these metabolites relative to in vivo concentrations, no predications regarding the potential for amphetamine or its metabolites to inhibit the metabolism of other drugs by CYP isozymes in vivo **can be** made.

~

With **normal** urine pHs approximately half of an

2. The Abnormal Orgasm

The stress of everyday life
usually does require treatment

Must balance risk
Need changes in behavior
Weak, no affinity
Exposure to people not important

Adjustment poor
Compared to normal subjects
Compared to normal subjects
Compared to *normal* subjects

Adjustment is necessary
Better than anxiety
Melancholia more effective
Significantly more effective

Fear of social situations
Exposure to unfamiliar people
The abnormal orgasm
The abnormal orgasm should be treated

The abnormal orgasm rate, less than 2 per minute,
was associated with a major increase following
therapy with alcohol, activated charcoal,
and a spoonful of applesauce.

Source: Package insert for Effexor (venlaraxine, an antidepressant)

patients and at a rate at least twice that of the placebo group for 4 placebo-controlled trials for **the** panic disorder indication (Table 6): gastrointestinal

~

Special Senses
Abnormal Vision5

~

8 Mostly "delayed **orgasm**" or "anorgasmia."

~

1 Adverse events for which the Effexor XR reporting **rate** was **less than** or equal to the placebo rate are not included. These events are: abdominal pain, accidental injury, anxiety, back pain,

~

disorder trials was associated with a mean final on-therapy increase in pulse rate of approximately **2** beats **per minute**, compared with 1 beat per minute for placebo. Effexor XR treatment for up to 8 weeks in premarketing placebo-controlled GAD trials **was associated with a** mean final on-therapy increase in pulse rate of

~

Effexor XR (venlafaxine hydrochloride) extended-release capsules treatment for up to 12 weeks in premarketing placebo-controlled trials for **major** depressive disorder was associated with a mean final on-therapy **increase** in serum cholesterol concentration of approximately 1.5 mg/dL

~

Events are further categorized by body system and listed in order of decreasing frequency using the **following** definitions:

~

thromboplastin time, or INR when venlafaxine was given to patients receiving warfarin **therapy.**

~

Among the patients included in the premarketing evaluation of Effexor XR, there were 2 reports of acute overdosage **with** Effexor XR in major depressive disorder trials, either alone or in

~

of acute overdose with venlafaxine, either alone or in combination with other drugs and/or **alcohol.** The majority of the reports involve

3. Kiddie Kare for Kops—Treatment of Children and Adolescents in ICE Compounds

COLORLESS WATER
exerts a beneficial effect.
SUPPRESSIVE ATTACKS IN THE FIELD
Children are especially sensitive to fatalities. A severe attack may be exacerbated. In these conditions the benefit outweighs the possible hazard.
PREGNANCY SHOULD BE AVOIDED
Radioactive mice passed rapidly across the placenta and accumulated in the eyes.
IMMEDIATE EVACUATION
may be effective, but artificial shock therapy may be forced to promote excretion of the parasite. In recent years certain strains have become resistant.
FAILING THE ENDEMIC ATTACK
may be calculated.
FOR RADICAL DISORDERS
who have not responded satisfactorily, irreversible damage has been observed. All should be questioned to detect any weakness. The unexplained should be regarded with suspicion.
DIFFERENT COMPOUNDS VARY
Emotional changes, nightmares, and atrophy of muscle may be associated with depression. Defects may progress. Weight loss is cumulative. The compound will require weeks to exert its beneficial effects. Film one face in a tight, light-resistant container.

Source: Package insert for Plaquenil (hydroxychloroquine, a cure for Covid-19. The best. What do you have to lose?)

Adverse effects with **different compounds vary** in type and frequency.

CNS Reactions: Irritability, nervousness, **emotional changes, nightmares**, psychosis,

~

progressive weakness **and atrophy of** proximal **muscle** groups which **may be associated with** mild sensory changes, **depression** of tendon reflexes and abnormal nerve conduction.

~

Visual field **defects**: Pericentral or paracentral scotoma, central scotoma, central scotoma

~

Retinopathy **may progress** even after the drug is discontinued. In a number of patients,

Rehearsal

I have started to practice my recollections.
This preparation will stand me in good stead.
Just as rehearsal enhances
the credibility of one's performance,
the efficient management of grief demands
a proper sorting and ranking of memories.
My most vivid memories
will consist of those occasions
when I could have treated you with greater kindness.

I have started to plan my wardrobe and makeup.
The former calls for clothes with a baggier fit,
reflecting inevitable loss of weight.
The latter requires little effort,
only slightly longer intervals
between haircuts, a few more days
of not shaving, and a general
indifference to how others see me.
I should adapt easily to concerted acts of neglect.

The greatest challenge of this role lies in
not knowing when the performance begins.
I'm the understudy for a part
I never auditioned to play.
You express irritation when I suggest a miracle
might occur or the playwright might amend the script.
You call this an absurd contrivance,
and I defer to your dramatic judgment.
I shall continue to rehearse.

Doctors Are Passing from Our Lives

~after Phillip Levine

When the administrator threatens our group
saying that our RVUs have fallen,
I riff on possible meanings of
the words Relative Value Unit.

Would it please him if I induced my cousin
and closest Relative, to come here for care?
His Medicaid wouldn't pay us shit,
but his complicated cirrhosis would generate a ton of RVUs.

As for Units, singularities, individual things,
we got that aced. One-of-a-kinds in this practice—
the unique, the sui generis, the once-in-a-lifetime—
are common as pennies.

Which leaves us with Value.
The regard we hold for something, its monetary worth,
perhaps its comparative worth relative to . . .
relative to . . . the price previously stated.

My colleagues start wadding their panties,
taking the administrator's implied threat more seriously than I.
They propose remedies ranging from advertising
to working longer hours to better parking

to merging with another group
to working longer hours
to shortening the time we spend with patients
to working longer hours.

[. . .]

The administrator believes we'll let him curl his claws
into our nostrils, carry us on his hip
like bowling balls, and send our heads
spinning down the lane. No. Not this doc.

GSW Chest

A lung desecrated by a bullet
spawns a perfect crimson bubble,
preternaturally stable, surface
galvanized by pulmonary proteins.
As these spheres blossom
between tension-torqued ribs,
coral foam flows
from mouth and nose
and makes it hard to apprehend
the victim's words, "Some dude."

Begin by sticking a tube into the pleural space,
and appreciate the paradox:
an assault on the chest
performed to treat
an assault on the chest.
Lots of blood coming out means a trip
to the OR stat, a consequence
surpassingly rare.
More commonly, merely watch
as the jar accumulates mostly air, some fluid.
Then call for the X ray.
While waiting—waiting way too long,
it always feels—for the radiology tech,
decide whether to
stick a breathing tube down
the throat. Expressions of gratitude
from the patient, if any,
can wait until later.

Wilfred Owen wrote of
blood *gargling* from lungs gassed,

[. . .]

or shredded by shrapnel,
or ripped by bayonets.
Not gurgling, no. Nor
bubbling, babbling, rippling, splashing.
Witness the victim's desperation,
his urge to clear his trachea
competing with the horror
of propelling more of his blood
into the blue plastic basin
thoughtfully placed beside his cheek by
an overworked nursing assistant.

You are witness now.
Write your barely legible prose.
In the box marked Diagnosis on
the urine-colored form, scribble "GSW Chest."

At last arrive at the hardest part.
Decide whether to open his chest or to observe.
Maybe the job is done,
no exploration required.
How close to the heart did the bullet pass as it went in?
How close as it traveled out?
How fast the pulse?
How low the pressure?
How oxygenated the finger or the earlobe?
Note the dragon tattoo, and
resolve to reassemble the beast
if a thoracotomy comes to pass.
Don't think of competing with Owen
or the ink of the anonymous artist.
Rather stick with the practical:
Operate now, at four a.m., when it's
easier to round up a scrub nurse, a first
assist, and an anesthesiologist?

Or watch, wait, and risk having to compete
with the OR's elective schedule.
With cases filling every slot
from dawn to late at night,
you'll have a devil of a time
getting an operating room at seven.
Best decide this minute.

Medical Marvels

It's tough sometimes in the heart unit
when things turn out completely different
from the way everyone initially expected.

Like the guy with chest pain
and a seriously bad looking echo study
who turned out to have merely nasty indigestion
from all the tacos and sangria he put away at lunch.

Or when the young girl who appeared
to have an ugly bacterial infection screwing
up her mitral valve actually suffered from an
extraterrestrial being taking possession of her heart,
a problem totally beyond my professional scope of practice.

Not that every unusual occurrence turns out so dramatic.
Sometimes a voodoo curse causes a rhythm disturbance,
and correcting the rhythm requires nothing more
than a reverse of the curse,
although given the paucity of voodoo consultants
in this neck of the woods,
that can take a week or even a month.

But our group takes pride in our management of infirmities
resulting from an unpleasant interaction
with figures from Greek mythology.
Medusa for instance.
When that bitch turns a person to stone, we jump into action
faster than wing-footed Hermes
and de-petrify the heart in minutes,
and we get the lungs and liver and other stuff
back in action almost as quickly, although to be honest,

we rarely get the knees and hips fully functional,
which is why you don't see our patients
playing full court basketball.

Emergency Room Nocturne

Before the pandemic
we took pride we knew the rules
for working the Saturday night shift
in the emergency room.

If a gunshot victim told us
the shooter was "some dude,"
he knew the name of the guy
who shot him and probably
had him on speed dial.

If he said that on a scale of one to ten,
the pain is a ten, we couldn't say it,
but we could think it.
"That must mean you're on fire.
And I don't see any flames."

If the patient's TTR—tattoo to tooth ratio—
was greater than two, he would survive
no matter what we did.

But rules don't apply since the virus.
Now the shooter can be anyone.
Now the bullets can't be seen.
Now we can catch one on the ricochet.

We used to patrol this arena
wearing only scrubs, fearing
only blood-borne invaders.
Now we dress like astronauts,
the ICU is full, and we have
refrigerated trucks because the
morgue can't hold all the bodies.

You know things are fucked
when *shortness of breath*
gets you sent home with an inhaler,
and we just ran out of inhalers.

We used to say the ER gets hit the worst
on Saturday nights with a full moon.
Now every night gets hit the worst.

Peonies

I remember asking the doctor whether the bleeding would ever stop.
I remember her telling me that all bleeding stops.

I remember how angry you became when the nurse asked
how you were,
    and you saying *as delighted as most people with this diagnosis,*
    and you asking the doctor about your odds of living one year,
    five years, ten,
    and you insisting *you better never call me a "survivor,"*
    and you demanding *you better never shave* your *head.*

I remember you telling me each of us stands alone, our bodies
mysteries of cyan spheres
    and auburn lights that gleam from haunted houses.
I remember thinking that was the chemo talking,
    and if that was the chemo talking, the chemo possessed greater
    eloquence than I would have expected.

I remember the night you estimated how many times I told you
I loved you.
I remember how you loved peonies, like the peonies I planted
on your grave.
I never told you I loved you often enough, I remember that too.

I remember you asking what were the odds of achieving immortality,
    and your reasoning that if you might drop dead tomorrow,
    cosmological symmetry decreed that you might also live forever.
I remember the importance you attached to cosmological
    symmetry.

I remember when the doctor said she needed to tighten up your
glucose,

and you began to sing "Tighten Up" by Archie Bell and the Drells,
and the other patients in the chemo room clapped along,
and you encouraged me to dance,
and I said that I was not a Drell, that the way I danced made me
the opposite of a Drell.

How I remember your silhouette backlit against the monitor's
orange glow,
and the burnt umber scrap of blanket artfully arranged to hide
the canister collecting all the bleeding that the doctor promised
would eventually stop.

I remember the doctor telling me that all bleeding stops.
I said that isn't exactly what I wanted to hear.
She said that isn't exactly what I wanted to tell you.

We Share What We Exhale

Oscar Wilde said give a man a mask.
And he will speak the truth.
What Wilde didn't say:
He will *hear* the truth.
A mask can barrier a virus, but
it can't prevent a lie from poisoning your ears.
You swallowed chloroquine.
You swallowed Clorox.
You swallowed bullshit more toxic
than either of those.

Because you refused to mask your face,
I must now mask mine.
I need to wear this fucker for two
or three or four hours
while I open up your chest,
because you couldn't wear one
for fifteen minutes
while you shopped at Costco
for your ten-pound bag of Funyuns.

This mask means no more to me
than the five thousand that came before
or the couple of hundred I have yet to put on.
Simon's mask might mean more to him,
because the hospital grudges the orderly just
one for his entire twelve hour shift.
Simon saddles up his mask sin tight before he dead lifts
your idiot carcass onto the operating table, with you
still awake,
still breathing on your own,
still capable of gahacking your pestilence
into Simon's face.

You needn't worry
that I will vent any of this in your direction.
I deem it unprofessional and inappropriate
to tattoo you with a political discussion
given the imbalance of the power relationship between you
and me, the one who unfumbles your heart with his hands.

Since I started this tirade with Wilde,
I shall close it appealing to Sontag,
who disdained the idea of illness as metaphor,
who rejected the concept of character
as determinant of disease.
Maybe Sontag, just this once,
would make an exception
for you.

Noise

It feels like it occurred during the Pleistocene,
but it was only a few decades ago that my
intern Brian taught me, a med student on my
first surgery rotation, the proper way to refer
to the Chief Complaint, the first and most
important component of a patient's history
and the basis for everything we do—
all the tests and the probes and the pokes
and the drugs and the scans and the operations—
that we might inflict on our fellow human being.

"What's his noise?" Brian asked.
"Chest pain," I said.
It filled me with inordinate pride
that Brian made an approving nod,
alleviating my own chest pain.

In a matter of days, all my fellow
third-year medical students adopted
the nomenclature, with chest pain a
a kind of *noise* and belly pain
a kind of *noise* and weak and dizzy
a kind of *noise* and getting hit by a streetcar
a kind of *noise* and getting shot
by a cop or by a friend or by some dude
a manifestation of *noise*.

The concept of *noise* expanded.
Our complaints about the cafeteria
constituted *noise* and grumbling about getting
hassled over overdue library books
constituted *noise* and bemoaning

when the city failed to clear the snow
and cars slid all over the streets
constituted *noise*.

Years passed, and arguments with spouses
created *noise* and professional frustrations
generated *noise* and financial difficulties—
although not all that difficult compared
to most people—offered consistent, reliable,
inevitable sources of *noise*.

All this is to say that as you sit here
in my office, and I ask you with warmth
and sincerity and compassion "What
brings you here today?" what I'm
really thinking is *What's your noise?*

I Worry

every time I enter the operating room
whether I made the correct diagnosis,
whether I planned the proper operation,
whether this 81-year-old man can endure the procedure.
Those are the easy ones.

I worry about the other members of my team.
Is my first assistant concentrating on this case,
or on whether we'll finish fast enough
that she can pick up her kid after school?
Has my anesthesiologist's focus faltered
because the hospital's administrators threaten
to outsource his specialty to a private equity firm?
I worry about myself, am I paying total attention
to this double valve replacement,
suppressing all thoughts about the lump
my wife will have biopsied tomorrow?

Over thirty-five years, the list lengthens:
An electrical failure, immersing us in darkness
save for my battery-powered headlight.
A contaminated blood transfusion,
dooming the patient years from now.
A housefly, designs malign,
buzzing through the room,
airlifting a sinister brigade of bacteria.

I learned to worry about earthquakes
after one rattled my operating room
like a properly shaken martini
minutes after I opened the baby's chest
but before I could get her
on the heart-lung machine.

But in all that time I never worried
whether a bomb would fall on me, a bomb
paid for by American taxes,
donated by an American president,
guided by American military intelligence,
the way bombs fell
on Dr. Hammam Alloh
on Dr. Medhat Saiham
on Dr. Ayman Abu al-Ouf,
and the way they continue to fall.

After Today

"After today," one of my partners asks me,
"What are you going to do?" He means,
what am I going to do in retirement after 35 years.
I tell him, "Something worthwhile.
Just to shake things up."
He laughs, but that's a question for tomorrow.

Today, I reflect that I got it wrong.
I thought I spent all these years holding
those hearts in my hands. But it was
those hearts holding on to me.

Today, for the final time, I don
blue-gray scrubs, sun-bright headlight,
three-point-five power optical loupes,
comfy sneakers consecrated by the
blood of thousands of patients and
permanently stained despite countless washings.

Today, I enter the operating room where
my scrub tech has opened her trays and aligned my tools
like knights on horseback ready to lay siege—
scalpels and rongeurs, scissors and trochars,
needles and lancets and osteotomes,
instruments machined from nickel and steel and titanium,
chrome and copper and lead—all the precious metals—
each instrument imparting its unique gratification when I grasp it,
when I touch it to the patient's heart.

Today, I await the arrival of my last patient,
who will lie on my operating table,
this marvel of ergonomic perfection

that adjusts smoothly, remains immobile,
and resists vibration when someone bangs into it.

After today, if I show up
in this room again,
I will be the one lying on this table.

ACKNOWLEDGMENTS

With gratitude to the editors of the following publications in which these poems originally appeared, some in slightly altered form.

december: "Doctor Ruiz didn't quit his job today"

Medmic: "GSW Chest"

Neon: "Rehearsal"

Sheila-Na-Gig: "Rejection Speech"

The AutoEthnologist: "Operating Theater," "Samuel L. Jackson Pulls a Shift in the Intensive Care Unit," "After Today," and "The Anatomy Lesson of Dr. Nicolaeus Tulp"

Unlost Journal: "Black Box Trilogy"

Writers Resist: "Velocity Squared"

EARLY PRAISE

"I read *The Pronunciation Part* in one sitting the first time around. Now, a few months later, I have read it straight through again, and with the same amazement and pleasure. These poems have the propulsive force of a page-turning novel coupled with accurate, edgy language that lends wit to even the grimmest situations. The poems are so vivid, I can see the chapbook as a short film. There is a historical line of physician literary artists. With *The Pronunciation Part,* Flavian Mark Lupinetti joins the tradition."

—Donna Hilbert, contest judge
author of *Threnody* and *Enormous Blue Umbrella*

Tough, a master storyteller, irreverent with a biting ironic sense of humor, a scalpel sharp intellect and deep compassion to match, Mark Lupinetti is a rare poet. This debut collection, *The Pronunciation Part,* opens onto a world readers of poetry seldom see, the world of a heart surgeon who performed decades of heart transplants and surgeries as well as worked in a hospital ER helping patients who ranged from pandemic Covid patients to gunshot victims. Who is more qualified to be a poet than a heart surgeon? The best poets are always heart surgeons resurrecting our hearts. Mark Lupinetti is a stunning example. Particularly moving is his poem, "Peonies" for his wife who died of cancer: *I remember the night you estimated how many times I told you I loved you./I remember how you loved peonies, like the peonies I planted on your grave.* From the first poem to the last, Lupinetti held me in his electric language thrall, with his unforgettable, impeccably crafted imagery where every single end line was a gut punch.

—Pamela Uschuk, author of *Refugee*
and *Crazy Love*, American Book Award

Crafting lived experience into thoughtful, compelling art is one of the things a poet can do, and exactly what Mark Lupinetti does in *The Pronunciation Part*. The poems in this chapbook are narrative driven, cohesive and have a tight-fisted muscularity to them, not unlike the human heart. Lupinetti's work makes the political intricately personal and thoroughly felt.

—**Elizabeth Jacobson author**
of *Not into the Blossoms* and *Not into the Air*

These poems align the practices of medicine and the lyric imagination, exploring the complexities, limits and revelations of both getting it right and getting it wrong. Only a perspective hard-won from decades in the operating room, and in the mind's operating room, could devastate and console with passages like *the only clue the patient has/ about the quality of the surgery/ is how well you closed the skin,* as in "Surgery Interns Know the Rules." I admire this excellent collection of poems.

—**Ed Skoog, author of *Mister Skylight,***
Rough Day* and *Travelers Leaving for the City

ABOUT THE AUTHOR

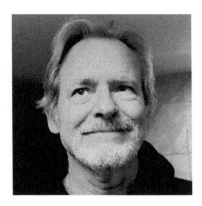

Flavian Mark Lupinetti, a Pushcart nominated poet, fiction writer, and cardiac surgeon, received his MFA from the Vermont College of Fine Arts. He received first place awards in the 2023 Social Justice Poetry Contest sponsored by *Sport Literate* and the 2014 Betsy Sholl Poetry Award sponsored by *Words and Images*. His creative writing has appeared in *Bellevue Literary Review, Cutthroat, december, Redivider, ZYZZYVA,* and other publications, and his contributions to the scientific literature include more than 90 peer-reviewed papers, research studies, and monographs. A native of West Virginia, Mark now lives in New Mexico.

About The Poetry Box® Chapbook Prize

The Poetry Box® Chapbook Prize is open to both established poets and emerging talent alike. The contest is open to poets residing in the United States and opens for submissions each year in February. Find more information at ThePoetryBox.com.

2024 Winners

The Pronunciation Part by Flavian Mark Lupinetti

Ice Cream for Lunch: A Grandparents Handbook by Laura Foley

A Girl, Her Slipper, and Yesterday's Rainbow by Allison Thorpe

2023 Winners

The Squannacook at Dawn by Richard Jordan

Inside Out by Kirsten Morgan

Reading Wind by Carol Barrett

2022 Winners

Tracking the Fox by Rosalie Sanara Petrouske

Elemental Things by Michael S. Glaser

Listening in the Dark by Suzy Harris

2021 Winners

Erasures of My Coming Out (Letter) by Mary Warren Foulk

Of the Forest by Linda Ferguson

Let's Hear It for the Horses by Tricia Knoll

2020 Winners

The Day of My First Driving Lesson by Tiel Aisha Ansari

My Mother Never Died Before by Marcia B. Loughran

Off Coldwater Canyon by C.W. Emerson

2019 Winners

Moroccan Holiday by Lauren Tivey

Hello, Darling by Christine Higgins

Falling into the River by Debbie Hall

2018 Winners

Shrinking Bones by Judy K. Mosher

November Quilt by Penelope Scambly Schott

14: Antología del Sonoran by Christopher Bogart

Fireweed by Gudrun Bortman

www.ingramcontent.com/pod-product-compliance
Lightning Source LLC
Chambersburg PA
CBHW060250060125
19918CB00007B/18